THE AIMS AND METHODS
OF MEDICAL SCIENCE

THE
AIMS AND METHODS OF
MEDICAL SCIENCE

An Inaugural Lecture

BY

JOHN A. RYLE

M.A., M.D., F.R.C.P.

Regius Professor of Physic in the University of
Cambridge, Consulting Physician to
Guy's Hospital, London

CAMBRIDGE
AT THE UNIVERSITY PRESS
1935

CAMBRIDGE
UNIVERSITY PRESS

University Printing House, Cambridge CB2 8BS, United Kingdom

Published in the United States of America by Cambridge University Press, New York

Cambridge University Press is part of the University of Cambridge.

It furthers the University's mission by disseminating knowledge in the pursuit of
education, learning and research at the highest international levels of excellence.

www.cambridge.org
Information on this title: www.cambridge.org/9781107656116

© Cambridge University Press 1935

First published 1935
Re-issued 2014

A catalogue record for this publication is available from the British Library

ISBN 978-1-107-65611-6 Paperback

THE AIMS AND METHODS
OF MEDICAL SCIENCE

It is not an easy moment nor an unembarrassed mood that brings me here—a stranger almost in the University of Cambridge, although the strangeness is already mitigated by much friendliness and welcome—to deliver my inaugural lecture. I have none of the advantages which my predecessors enjoyed in the shape of early training in this school or other bonds and associations with the University. Of the high traditions of your medical faculty I have, in common with the rest of my profession, had ample and frequent testimony, but your systems and your customs and the atmosphere of your life I have yet to learn.

The mood and the moment are lacking in ease not only because I am a newcomer, but also because I must inevitably make comparisons in the matter of endowments between myself and those who have gone before me. These have been men of a scholarly distinction to which I cannot lay claim and of a professional seniority, which time alone can add to me. They have set a high standard that must needs implant humility in any successor. I am, however, so much indebted, in one way and another, to my three immediate predecessors, and two of them have given me such generous exhortation and counsel, that I take courage and inspiration from them and face the future with an eager determination to give, as they did, all that I can of service to Cambridge medicine. For the gifts and prospects which Cambridge offers me I shall hope that London and the school of Guy's may, through my endeavours, make just return.

Sir Clifford Allbutt I did not know personally, but to his literary culture, to his writings on arterial disease and angina pectoris in particular, and to his historical and educational essays I have long been in debt. Sir Humphry Rolleston, from the moment when I first met him in the examination hall to the present day, has shown me frequent kindnesses. Many of his erudite contributions to the science and art of medicine I have admired and treasured. His biography of Clifford Allbutt, a parting gift from my friend and colleague Dr Arthur Hurst, and his history of the Cambridge Medical School, have been my companions in recent weeks. From Sir Walter Langdon Brown's writings I have also drawn frequent benefits. He and I have had some of our happiest associations in connection with a small club, consisting of a group of London physicians, which meets informally at the end of laborious days to discuss the problems of clinical medicine and clinical education in their broadest sense, always with refreshment and sometimes with inspiration to the minds of its members. He too has shown me constant kindness on the eve of my present appointment.

The Scope and present Shortcomings of Medical Science

I have chosen to discuss, in a very general way, the aims and methods of Medical Science, and to indulge both in criticism and a forecast. It seemed to me a suitable moment for such a survey, for I am leaving one field of activity, or rather of many activities, for duties of a new kind and more directly and whole-heartedly

7

concerned (although much of my time has already been devoted to teaching and study) with the advancement of medical learning. The aims of medical science may be briefly and broadly stated. They are to increase and perfect our knowledge (with a view to its control) of disease in man, and equally our knowledge of man in disease, by every legitimate means of science and art at our disposal. In furtherance of this aim the study of healthy structure and function play a leading part. Close clinical observation and accurate recording of the living phenomena of disease; the evaluation of environmental and hereditary factors; morbid anatomy and histology; the study of the chemical and bacterial agents of disease and of immunity; psychology; biochemistry; radiology; pharmacology; dietetics; and the experimental production of disease in animals, provide the principal methods whereby the solution of our problems is sought. Observation and experiment are, or should be, equal partners in our scheme.

Within the profession only those few have lost sight of the aims of medical science who have made a trade of their art, or who, through some combination of mental peculiarity and faulty education, indulge in cranks or succumb to the fixed idea, basing their actions upon methods which have no true relationship with what is generally understood by scientific method. We must admit, however, that even among the vast body of honest workers who have the proper aims in view (and I refer here both to practitioners and laboratory men) there remains too great a proportion whose standards of accuracy, whose use of evidence and whose critical faculties are defective, whose judgment is continually crippled, rather than gradually amended, by the inherent difficulties of their subject and the exacting conditions of their lives. The objects of their task are more or less apparent to them, but their use of the tools which they bring to it is clumsy or the tools themselves are inappropriate.

To what primary errors are these shortcomings due? Firstly, we have not been strict enough in our selection of men, whether by elimination of unsuitable students at an early stage in their career, or by direction of energies into proper channels after qualification. Secondly, our systems of education and examination—although reforms are pending—have become too complicated and unwieldy, our instruction too uncorrelated and departmental, too insistent on the acquisition of knowledge without provision for its proper distribution and assimilation. Thirdly, we have allowed the cult of specialism, both in clinical and laboratory work, and in the training for these, to spread unchecked and have lost sight of the need for a central controlling philosophy to hold the reins of the restive younger sciences.

With the first two errors I am not here concerned, but, as few days go by in my professional life in which I do not behold faulty judgments due to lack of vision or to that inaccurate focussing of vision which is the outcome of too much specialism, I shall ask leave to consider the third in closer detail.

The Defects of Specialism

In all that I say please believe that I am not condemning specialism as such, for good specialism is essential to all scientific progress. I condemn only excessive, premature and misdirected specialisms for the subversive influences which they have had upon medical thought and action and education. There is an element of truth in the facetious dictum which describes the specialist as one "who knows more and more about less and less", but my present attitude is better expressed by a phrase of Hughlings Jackson, who said: "There is no harm in studying a special subject; the harm is in doing any kind of work with a narrow aim and a narrow mind." He was himself pleading for better integration in the sciences as a counterpart to increasing specialisation.

We should also remind ourselves that, while specialism in medicine can often deliver new truths or refinements of old truths, it can rarely of itself, in the complex human problems which confront us, give anything approaching the whole truth about a patient or his disease.

Now a teacher of general medicine and a consultant in general medicine has peculiar opportunities of observing errors which result from the causes which I seek to define. He rubs shoulders continually with students, practitioners, clinical specialists and scientists and, last but not least, with patients of all degrees, and acquires in the process some familiarity with the needs and problems of them all. He may, perhaps, fall himself into the "specialism" of being "too general" in his opinions, but his functions are essentially judicial and he is continually in the position of having to balance the opinions and evidence of others. The science and art of medicine are more constantly complementary in his particular work than in the work of the general practitioner, the surgical or medical specialist or the whole-time professor. Philosophy, psychology and scientific thought make common cause in his daily affairs, although he separately professes none of them.

I should be the last to pretend to infallibility of judgment in matters clinical, but, mingled with countless examples of good and wise industry, my practice has brought all too frequently before me instances of operations unnecessarily undertaken or advised, of treatments injudiciously selected and forecasts unfairly given, not because of the inherent difficulties of medicine which tax us all, but simply because the nature and meaning of common symptoms have been insufficiently appreciated; because new machines and tests have been allowed to usurp the function of eye, or ear, or hand, or native wit; because the psychology of a patient has been misread or neglected in the previous estimates; or because he or she has never been viewed as a "whole" man or woman, and the disease never studied as a "whole" disease. All too commonly the puzzled practitioner has been persuaded into unwise diagnosis or action by a laboratory or radiological opinion unjustified because it has been given without reference to or knowledge of the general situation, which includes both organism and environment, part and whole. In an earlier generation deficiencies in the matter of precise tests and scientific detail were often compensated for by close observation and the applications of a sane logic. The educations of to-day leave little room for the training of reason. They pile up evidence but neglect instruction in its use. This tendency to inco-ordinate action is still growing and can be corrected only by a return to first principles.

General Smuts, in his philosophical discourse entitled "Holism and Evolution", has critically considered this tendency to continued sub-division of knowledge in Science and the disadvantages which have accrued and continue to accrue therefrom. Other sciences besides Medicine have suffered from the abandonment of what Bacon called universality or *philosophia prima*. Writing on this theme in *The Advancement of Learning* he says: "Another error...is the over early and peremptory reduction of knowledge into arts and methods; from which time commonly sciences receive small or no augmentation. But as young men, when they knit and shape perfectly, do seldom grow to a further stature; so knowledge, while it is in aphorisms and observations, it is in growth; but when it once is comprehended in exact methods, it may perchance be further polished and illustrate and accommodate for use and practice; but it increaseth no more in bulk and substance."

If we leave the field of practice for the field of laboratory enquiry and research we are confronted with the same disturbing tendencies. Throughout the world there are (to take a single instance) earnest men, both young and old, researching into cancer who never see a case of cancer from one year's end to the other and, often enough, have but the smallest contacts with those who see the cases and the living disease and observe the variations in its course and the individual peculiarities of its victims. It may be said that such contacts are not necessary and that results are produced without them and that, for all his small therapeutic triumphs, nothing has been more helpless than the attitude of the clinician in the face of cancer, but it is not the experience of the past that great advances are ever made without the attack on the broad front or close co-operation of all arms in the attack.

The bacteriologist studies the agents of disease, but only occasionally sees the disease or its consequences in the living or even in the defunct patient. If he does so it is in the moment of taking his specimen of blood or body-fluid and often without a proper interest in the whole event. In the case of the bacteriologist who seeks to assist directly in the treatment of disease this abstraction from it has resulted in graver evils. Until lately it has been a common experience of consulting practice to find that a bacteriologist (a man whose training is presumed to be far more scientific than that of the physician) has been willing to prescribe treatment in the shape of a vaccine, prepared from a throat-swabbing or a faecal specimen, for a patient whom he has never seen and who has had no precise diagnostic label assigned to him, and without any evidence that there existed a causal relationship between the organisms isolated and the patient's malady, or that a vaccine can produce the response it is supposed to produce. I could wish that some of the less balanced but more assertive bacteriologists of this country could borrow the humility of an Indian colleague from whom I recently received a sheaf of reports with the following cautious foot-note attached to each: "This report carries a no-guarantee. God alone is infallible."

As examples of miscarriage of medical justice, but with the blame divided between clinician and bacteriologist, I have seen gout treated as rheumatoid arthritis, phthisis treated as bronchitis, and symptoms due to the abuse of purgatives treated as colitis for long periods with vaccines. The criticisms with which Clifford Allbutt teased the gynaeco-logists in his Goulstonian Lectures fifty years ago could be multiplied for every specialism which has since evolved. Nevertheless Medi-cine owes an incalculable debt to these same specialisms; my censure is of those who bring discredit on them and of our educational systems.

We are to-day training numbers of young and enthusiastic biochemists to help in the investigation of new and old problems; theirs is a branch of medical science full of promise for the future, but the arrangements for them are often such that they will not grow up in the appreciation of what the living problems are, nor share sufficiently with the clinical workers the difficulties which both of them are anxious to resolve. There is a danger that the less able and the less fortunately placed among them may drift as the less favoured bacteriologists have drifted and bring disservice instead of benefits to their own science and to medicine as a whole. Even without this it seems to me that the constant partition of their enquiries must often detach their thought and actions from essential problems.

Specialisation on the part of those responsible for the education of the student, both in the clinical and the pre-clinical periods, also grows apace, and it is small wonder that in the final year we meet with diffuse and bewildered minds.

The general physiologist and the general pathologist have conferred incalculable benefits on medicine directly by their original work and indirectly by their education of the student, but as the general physician is becoming rare through the drift towards early specialisation, so too, it seems to me, a similar drift is threatening their sciences. It is already becoming difficult to fill the chairs of physiology and pathology in the London medical schools with men of suitably broad education and attainments.

Where there is progressive segregation and subdivision of research, co-operation between services becomes less easy and more rare. The physician and the physiologist have innumerable common interests, but they work in isolation one from the other. Subjective symptoms are a main concern of the physician; they proclaim for the most part disturbances, whether in the direction of exaggeration or depression, of normal reflex activity or other vital phenomena. They are specific, not for diseases, but for physiological error due sometimes to a variety of causes. They are eminently deserving of closer study; but the physiologist does not see and, in animals, can rarely reproduce the symptoms, while the physician has not the time or training to enable him to investigate them otherwise than by observational and inductive methods. Again the physician has gathered much information to suggest that predisposition to many disease-states is to be found in inborn biological variations—sometimes called diatheses. Ignorance of normal variability has been a cause of much wrong diagnosis and treatment. Few things have helped my own orientation more than an early enquiry which revealed to me the extremes of motor and secretory activity of the healthy stomach. The study of anatomical and physiological variability in health might yet provide a fruitful field of enquiry for the anatomist and physiologist with valuable reflections for clinical science.

Everywhere around us we see the men and the will and the work, but too rarely the opportunity and the contacts needful for achievement. We know the aims but lack the method. Healthy and well-directed and correlated specialism is and will remain the life-breath of science, but the waste of time and monies in the world through the drive towards isolated, pigeon-holed research on the part of young men whose education has lacked breadth from the beginning and the very nature of whose appointments and whose tasks deprives them of the stimulus they most need, is to me a sad thought. The divorce of ward from laboratory is still in large part to blame.

The Lessons of Achievement

Nevertheless we are, from time to time, refreshed by far-reaching advances in our knowledge. It should then be pertinent to enquire into the factors which have favoured success. Is it not commonly the case that the clinician has made himself his own experimentalist, or *vice versa*—in the past it was so with Harvey, Jenner and Lister—or that the collaboration between experimentalist and clinician has been so close and intimate that they may almost be said to have worked with one mind?

It has been proper of late to cite as outstanding examples of new medical progress the important contributions of men like Sir Frederick Banting and Professor Minot. Banting, a young clinician, conceived an idea. With the help of his friend Best and his physiological mentor, Professor MacLeod, he put the idea to the test of experiment and obtained his proofs. It was not long before his claims were happily substantiated at the bed-side. Minot and his collaborators went through a similar process in discovering the treatment which has provided the answer to pernicious anaemia, and incidentally initiated a fruitful enquiry into the problems of haemopoiesis and the pathology and therapeutics of the anaemias generally. Sir Patrick Laidlaw, although his work is confined to the laboratory, and the animal-house, setting himself the severest conditions and meticulous about his controls, has made brilliant contributions in the case of distemper and influenza, largely because he has appointed himself his own animal doctor and the natural historian of their diseases. He sees and superintends the whole of his experiment; *materies morbi*, patients, autopsies are all in his and his assistants' hands. Sir Thomas Lewis, pursuing other problems, has brought precise experimental methods to the bed-side, setting a fine example to all who have a love of clinical accuracy and a desire for new clinical truths.

Nearly twenty years ago it fell to me to be a

partner in a very complete and happy piece of work, the fruitful results of which were largely due to the fact that the master-mind of the pathologist who was responsible for it was interested throughout in the patients, the disease as a whole, its morbid anatomy and histology, the agents of the disease, its epidemiology, and its reproduction in animals. I refer to the investigation of Spirochaetal Jaundice (Weil's Disease) in Flanders during the War by my friend Adrian Stokes, later to die of Yellow Fever in West Africa. In this investigation W. H. Tytler and I were privileged to play a part. We lived in the same mess. Stokes was in my ward and I was in his laboratory day by day. He saw my cases. I saw his guinea-pigs. He had a "spot-map" made of infected trenches and secured rats from them. The same disease was produced in rat-inoculated as in man-inoculated guinea-pigs. A rat-infected guinea-pig was protected by a convalescent soldier's serum. Non-icteric cases were recognised. The disease in man and the experimental animal were critically compared. We kept our study whole;

we shared our observations; our material and work were concentrated in one place. Results and proofs followed. Admittedly Stokes—a rare and eager spirit—was in command and the opportunities were favourable, but problem-sharing was perfected in a manner which rarely obtains under existing conditions.

Could not lessons of the kind I have quoted be more frequently applied? Where should they best find their application? It might be supposed that the large city hospitals with their abundant clinical material would furnish the best opportunities. In fact, however, the conditions of staffing, the multiple duties and the necessary routine which fall to the various members both of the clinical and laboratory staffs, and the dependence of the clinician on private practice for his livelihood make any form of team-work or close collaboration extremely difficult. The appointment of whole-time research physicians advocated by Sir Thomas Lewis and already supported by the Medical Research Council will shortly, no doubt, bear fruit, but intimate co-operation with the other scientific departments will usually remain an essential and will not always be easy of consummation. We must be careful lest we isolate yet another specialism. The methods of discovering and training research physicians may also need to be modified from time to time. An early and intensive experimental training cannot compensate for or provide the stimulus derived from daily contacts with a rich variety of cases.

Clinical Science as a University Subject

There remains the University with a flourishing medical faculty and a well equipped hospital at hand. Here again Sir Thomas Lewis, ever fruitful of ideas and eager for his own science, has, in his recent Huxley Lecture, visualised the recognition of Clinical Science as a University subject and the establishment of clinical units within the University. And surely, where we have assembled in one place the best anatomists, physiologists, pathologists and biochemists and the finest facilities for teaching and research, it is only reasonable to suggest that the circuit should, in due course, be completed by an active

Department of Clinical Medicine. That such a department (while capable of supplying illustration and demonstration) should not be destined primarily for the training of under-graduate students, whose numbers and whose needs make it imperative that they should continue to seek the prolific and varied material and experience of the London hospitals, is evident. But that research into human biology in its widest aspects, into the biology of man in health and disease, should continue in the absence of patients and diseases to study and of persons equipped for their study, is surely something of an anomaly. Such a department would gain greatly from its contacts with the other scientific departments of the University, and should have benefits to confer on them in return.

Given beds, an out-patient clinic and a laboratory, it should be capable of employing continually a small selected group of young qualified men and training them in the best methods of clinical observation and research. As the departments of Physiology, Anatomy, Pathology and Biochemistry are largely concerned with training recruits for their sciences, so also would a Department of Clinical Medicine be largely concerned with the training of physicians by the provision of opportunity, guidance and material. A certain number of beds would need to be set aside for particular studies under the supervision of the head of the Department, but as much clinical material as possible, and material of every kind, should be available for his assistants, who might well act simultaneously as assistants to the members of the visiting staff and as liaison officers between the Clinical Department and the other departments of the University. In this way and with inter-departmental conferences a better unity of interest and purpose might well be realised.

It would take too long to enumerate the possible interests and functions of such a department, but the study of symptoms, their nature and their purpose, by more precise methods, would be a main consideration.* Intensive and continuous study of common

* Whatever may be done in the future in the way of disease-prevention by improved hygiene, dietetics

27

diseases should generally be preferred to isolated research on rare ones. Therapeutic trials and the early disproof by experiment of the extravagant claims which are made from time to time on behalf of new tests and treatments, at present so liable to distort professional reason and opinion and to bring discredit upon medicine, might constitute a practical service. The more accurate portraiture of diseases, improvements in diagnostic and prognostic methods, and studies of innate predisposition would provide appropriate tasks. A follow-up system should be an essential element of the scheme. Only thus can we learn the true natural history of disease and the effects of treatment. The services of the department to the hospital could only be stimulating and

and a better understanding of aetiology, we must also remember that there are many chronic diseases (such as peptic ulcer, bacilluria and the severe anaemias) which would not become chronic if the meaning of the subjective phenomena which herald them were more widely appreciated. Symptoms which Dr John Brown described as "the voice of nature" and "everywhere available" are still poorly attended to, and the constant search for new objective proofs has encouraged their neglect.

salutary, and there should be no artificial separation between its functions and those of the visiting and resident staffs, whose members would in fact complete the unit.

The physician, the student of φύσις or nature, as his name implies, is ideally the man who sees the problems and sees them whole. He is not always the man to separate and solve them in their details, but in a given case or a given disease he alone is, by his training, in a position to assess the contribution of the various factors at work and to indicate where specialist help is likely to prove of value. As the natural historian of disease he is concerned with its accurate delineation and classification and broader comprehension. At times, if given proper facilities, he may take to himself other methods of enquiry (for the naturalist may also be an experimental biologist) but minute and accurate observation and record, with careful comparisons and deductions, are his first contributions. He must remain something of an anatomist, a physiologist, a pathologist and especially a psychologist, and yet is none of these or only sufficiently so to give

29

him free access to the minds of the experts in these sciences. And yet he too has experience upon which all of these may draw. They study parts. His interest is the whole.

The Meaning of Clinical Science

Perhaps I may be allowed a digression here to consider what we are to understand by the term "Clinical Science", how far it is to be regarded as something separate from clinical medicine as a whole, and how far it embodies principles and methods distinct from those which physicians have customarily observed and employed. Sir Thomas Lewis has been at pains to explain his meaning of the term and I cannot do better than quote his words:

"This science", he says, "seeks by observation and otherwise, to define diseases as these occur in man; it attempts to understand these diseases and their many manifestations, and here especially makes frequent use of the experimental method. It makes definite experiments upon disease or watches the effects of experiments conducted by injuries, however these arise; it culls, or actually creates, and uses physiological or pathological knowledge

30

immediately related and applicable to the diseases studied. Its value has been abundantly and frequently displayed in this country by such experimental clinicians as Ferrier, Horsley, Mackenzie and Head. The very mention of these names is in effect a definition of the science that is in mind. Their work was not work that could be delegated to laboratories; it was inspired and sustained by direct contacts with disease; it was carried through in very large or chief measure by observations on sick people." (*Brit. Med. Journ.* 15th March, 1930.)

In his Huxley lecture he also makes reference to a similar view expressed long since by Sir James Paget, who said:

"I feel sure that clinical science has as good a claim to the name and rights and self-subsistence of a science as any other department of biology; and that in it are the safest and best means of increasing knowledge of diseases and their treatment...." "Receiving thankfully all the help that physiology or chemistry or any other sciences more advanced than ours can give, and pursuing all our studies with the precision and circumspection that we may best learn from them, let us still hold that, within our range of study, that alone is true which is proved clinically, and that which is clinically proved needs no other evidence."

Finally Lewis has indicated even more clearly in his book entitled *Clinical Science, illustrated by Personal Experiences* (London, 1934) the types of enquiry which exemplify his programme and beliefs.

While, however, he is careful to allow that all systematic studies of disease in living man, whether observational or experimental, are appropriate to Clinical Science, he would have us accept that future advancements (as with other sciences) will lie more and more in the department of experimentation, with the corollary that the contributions of observational medicine, having been so long tested and employed, are no longer likely to prove as profitable. Here I find myself less frankly in agreement with him, firstly because there are necessary and rather strict limits to the possibilities of experiment in the case of sick persons and because the types of disease which at present lend themselves to this kind of study are few in number; and secondly because, by more precise and intensive methods of observational study and the addition of new instruments and methods, I believe that our knowledge of man's ills can continue indefinitely to be usefully served and even, perhaps, as usefully served as by the experimental method. Lewis has been happy as well as wise in his selection of problems for study by clinical experiment. Cardio-vascular disease, pulse phenomena, the capillary circulation, the phenomena of Raynaud's disease, cutaneous reactions, the pain of intermittent claudication and the kindred pain of angina pectoris, are all in some degree adapted to experimental as well as observational study, and the experiments can be performed without harm and with little inconvenience to the patients. The symptoms of these diseases are commonly accompanied by visible or palpable and sometimes measurable phenomena of an objective kind. It is very difficult to think (although I may here lack ingenuity and foresight) of other types or groups of disease in which the conditions are as favourable. In the acute and chronic infections, in blood-diseases, digestive disorders, and respiratory diseases it is rarely possible to reproduce or vary or to measure symptoms at will. In diseases of the nervous system, excepting by surgical experiment, it is also difficult to imagine any form of research which can promise better increments to knowledge than the existing methods of constantly closer and more accurate studies of history and after-history, and of symptoms and signs, by recognised clinical methods and with the aid of such improvements as may be added to us by better instrumental and laboratory technique or supplied by physiological investigation in animals.

Humane considerations, as Lewis has insisted, must always set limits to clinical experiment, which can never be allowed to cause any hurt or to interfere with curative measures or relief of symptoms, even though we may, on occasion, be perfectly justified in endeavouring to examine a patient during the production of a symptom for purposes of better diagnosis and a more complete understanding of it. I have already voiced my contention (conscious of my debt in the matter to Hilton, Head, Mackenzie, Hurst and others) that the more accurate study of symptoms should open a rich field of research, but by observational study alone of the experiments which nature herself provides there is much still to be done. There is no bodily pain which might not be more closely analysed by simple methods of examination, interrogation and accurate record. Such analyses are surely scientific, even if, at present, they cannot include exact measurements. After all such biophysical and biochemical measurements as we are now able to make in the assessment of bodily function are only accurate in a relative sense, as we are frequently reminded by their variability in health and from time to time and case to case in comparable conditions of disease.

To revert to the study of an individual pain, our knowledge of it may be improved by considerations of its character, severity, situation, localisation or diffusion, paths of reference, duration, frequency, special times of occurrence, aggravating and relieving factors and associated symptoms and signs; by knowledge of the patient's psychological type and general state of physical health; and by correlative radiological, endoscopic or other studies of the painful organ or structure. There are very few pains which have been systematically studied in this way. Some of them, although rarely in the case of the more remote viscera, can be reproduced or imitated in healthy subjects. Hurst's enquiries into "The Sensibility of the Alimentary Canal" (Goulstonian Lectures, 1911) and Carlson's work on "The Control of Hunger in Health and Disease" afford notable examples of such researches.

I am also of the opinion that our knowledge can still be greatly improved by more accurate studies which seek to establish the true natural history of disease. Prognosis especially benefits and therapeutic ideas receive correction from such studies. The zoologist and the botanist and the geologist are not considered unscientific because they employ methods which differ from those of the physicist and chemist and because measurement and minute analyses are less appropriate to their tasks.

In a particular case or disease the physician has to consider such aetiological factors as age, sex, inheritance, temperament, physical type, environment, occupation, habits, and past illness, in addition to present symptoms, course and response to therapeutic agents. He has to assess whether improvements are due to natural repair or his own ministrations and to keep his mind very open in these decisions. Of pulse, respiration-rate, temperature and weight he must often keep accurate readings. Of the influence of the patient's psychology on his physical processes and *vice versa* he must be an attentive student. He must be alert to seize new opportunity when physiology, biochemistry, pathology or pharmacology present a fresh idea. He must seek correction whenever possible in the post-mortem room. By all these methods conscientiously applied and developed he advances his own and the general store of knowledge. He cannot afford not to be a student of the "whole". When possible he should certainly add clinical experiment to his scheme. He should train those entrusted to him—whatever researches they may undertake—to the belief that they must never do so to the neglect of old and tried routine. Huxley's definition of science as "trained and organised common-sense" has a special application to clinical science.

Integration and the Future

I have sought to show, what we all know in our hearts, that segregation and specialisation in medicine and the medical sciences have advanced too quickly; that we have lost what Bacon called *philosophia prima* and Smuts would call the "holistic" outlook; that there is need in practical medicine for a revival of interest in what Sir William Gull, one of the wisest physicians of the Guy's school, called "the general view"; and avoidance, as he phrased it, of "too narrow a pathology"; that in medical science the time for the task of integration, however difficult it may be, is overdue.

The rapid and influential developments of medicine in recent times have had the effect of deceiving both professional and lay minds into the belief that what derives from the laboratory is necessarily more scientific and nearer to the truth than what is observed at the bed-side. Utilising freely but relying too much on the test-tube or the contributions of radiology and instrumental device or despairing because of these of their own abilities, many doctors have lost their own souls (if the soul be compounded of or directed by the senses) and have failed to learn how profitably disease may be studied with eye and ear and hand and nose and the wit which garners essential information from the history, the environment, the relatives or friend. A bed-side or consulting-room analysis is often far more scientific in process and achievement than the summary of detached laboratory analyses which fill the dossier of the wealthy valetudinarian; even more scientific some-times than accredited publications in the journals of research. Properly conducted the examination of each patient is a simple exer-cise in biological enquiry. In practice we know our limitations and our great de-pendence in many circumstances upon the chemist, the pathologist and the radiologist, but without a proper sifting and synthesis of results their help is uncertain and their con-tributions may mislead. In other fields of biological research the need for co-ordination of methods is just as great. Observation and experiment are both essential, but they must go hand in hand. Both are capable of being scientifically or unscientifically used. The mind adapted for one is not always adapted for the other. The training in either case is a stern training. It is a main criticism of modern pre-clinical education that it does so little to foster the habit of observation. It is a main criticism of the later periods in the medical curriculum that they so readily allow the ideals of accuracy fostered by an experimental training to be lost to view.

I am hopeful enough, however, to believe that we shall see in the next decade or two a renaissance in Medicine, which will be marked by an eagerness on the part of the younger men (perhaps after a period in hospital or private practice, perhaps after a period of training in experimental method, for both have important lessons to give) to turn more frequently to the study of problems at the bed-side and with a greater care and accuracy than they have ever before been studied. A happier partition of problems and a closer collaboration between the ward and the laboratory, between students of normal and morbid physiology, than obtains at present will surely play their part.

Physiology and clinical medicine have a host of related problems. The clinician and the biochemist are eager for new associations. Pharmacology, which owes so much to laboratory experiment, still stands in need of better bed-side opportunity. The atmosphere of the University, free as it is of many of the distractions and difficulties which (for all the fine work accomplished therein) embarrass life and action in the city hospitals should be a healthy one for the growth of correlative studies, for the training of the scientific clinician (who, let me add, to be scientific and a discoverer must also be psychologically alert and watchfully humane), and for specialisation and integration to thrive together. Within the University we are concerned with science itself, the education for the pursuit of science and the preliminary education for the application of science to practice. In all of these departments it is our proper aim to employ and to train not narrow or diffuse but broad and organised intelligence.

Medicine needs again general physicians of the type of Sydenham, Heberden, Trousseau, Bright, Gull, Wilks, Osler and Allbutt to partner the able neurologists, cardiologists, pediatrists and psychiatrists and research physicians of our present age, and to "leaven the lump" of knowledge from which, through example and precept, through consultation and lectures and the journals, the whole profession derives no small part of its inspirations and its standards.

Physiology and pathology too need more general physiologists and pathologists to partner and direct their increasing progeny of specialised investigators. Among teachers, both clinical and pre-clinical, we require a fuller appreciation of the present difficulties and ultimate needs of the student; among research-workers a deeper sympathy with each other's tasks, a more naturalistic approach to many problems and a higher scale of philosophic values.

I may seem to commend too much my own subject—Clinical Medicine—but it is not a narrow one, and it has intimate associations with all the subjects that to-day come under the heading of Medical Science. You will therefore, I trust, bear with me when I urge that the ward, with its associate out-patient clinic and laboratories, must become once more both the starting and the rallying point of many researches, its problems the round table topics, as it were, for much corporate discussion and enterprise. The more minute and intimate study of the causes, the processes and the consequences of a disease must never be separated by too wide a gap in space or time from the study of the disease itself and the victims of the disease. The study of "wholes" and the study of "parts" must proceed in close conjunction. Does not the very word "University" imply provision for this comprehensive ideal?

How are the processes of synthesis and integration to be achieved? Firstly I believe, by ensuring the training of a sufficiency of students and teachers of the parent subjects, of workers in the general fields of Physiology, Pathology and Medicine; and secondly by improving the liaison between the ancillary and parent sciences and, perhaps, arranging for interchange of workers between the "clinical" and "scientific" services. Should we not remind ourselves that Clinical Medicine was the parent of them all, and that, for this reason and in virtue of its re-invigoration by scientific thought and method, its claims to equal partnership are just and salutary? There are, as I have sought to show, good reasons for desiring to see a better provision in our universities for the training of scientific physicians as well as medical scientists.

Only once before have I had the honour to address a Cambridge audience. At the invitation of the University Medical Society I then gave a dissertation on "The Physician as Naturalist". I should like to conclude my present remarks with a quotation from Bacon's "Advancement of Learning" which stood for my opening text on that occasion: "Only there is one thing still remaining, which is of more consequence than all the rest: namely, a true and active Natural Philosophy for the Science of Medicine to be built upon."

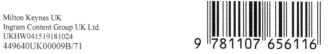